LEPTIN DIET

50
Days of Powerful Leptin Diet Recipes
to Boost Resistance,
Achieve Optimum Health
and Lose Weight Naturally

P. 12
55
17√

J. J. Lewis

Want more Bestseller Cook Books for **FREE?**

Join my **V.I.P** Reading List where I give away **Healthy** and Delicious
Recipes **FOR FREE!**

Yes, you heard me right! COMPLETELY FREE to everyone just for being a
loyal reader of mine!

www.ravenspress.com/jjlewis

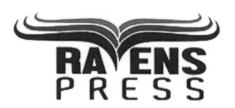

RAVENS PRESS

ISBN-13: 978-1516895052

ISBN-10: 1516895053

www.amazon.com/author/jjlewis

Table of Contents

Introduction

If you are reading this book, chances are that you or a loved one has been diagnosed with Leptin Resistance. Just like with any medical condition, the first and most important steps are to educate yourself on the disorder, learn its effects on the body, and then learn how to manage it.

Over 50 million people in the United States suffer from this disorder. This means that about one out of every six people are fighting against their own body and their own hormones in their efforts to lose weight and become healthier. They are also fighting a battle with diet and portion size. They are fighting with their body to control hunger cravings and the need to snack.

No matter how you look at it, your body sending signals of hunger all the time is just not fair to you. Your own body forcing you to eat, or telling you that unhealthy portion sizes are necessary for you to be comfortable is completely ridiculous, and only YOU can put a stop to it.

Within the pages of this book, you will develop a full understanding of Leptin Resistance, as well as strategies for controlling and reversing the resistance your body has built.

This guide provides information on how to holistically manage this disorder on a natural level and in combination with medications your doctor may prescribe.
I am here to tell you how to take control of your Leptin levels and your resistance, and to become a healthier, happier you that can stand proud.

Thank you for downloading this book. I hope you are able to develop a great understanding of Leptin Resistance and how to treat your body in a holistic manner to control the effects of this disorder on your body.

Chapter 1: What is Leptin?

Leptin is a protein hormone that regulates the expenditure and intake of energy in the body. Leptin plays a crucial part in the regulation of metabolism and appetite. The protein, Leptin, was discovered in the 1950's inside the Jackson Laboratory while studying mice with a homozygous obese (ob) mutation on its genetic strain. The researchers found that these mice were massively obese and ate excessive amounts of food.

By the 1960's, the researchers were able to typify the defective gene. It was only in the 1990's that the defective obese gene was mapped. By 1994, the ob gene was finally discovered and identified as the hormone leptin by Jeffrey Friedman. The term Leptin comes from the Greek word lepto, which means thin. This is because the normal allele of the ob gene keeps a person thin, unlike its mutant gene.

The Science Behind Leptin

In humans, the ob gene is found in chromosome 7 and is composed of 16 kDa adipose-driven proteins with a total of 167 amino acids.

Most of the leptin hormones are created within the body's white fat deposits; therefore, the amount of leptin within the body is directly connected with the body's total fat.

Leptin can also be created within brown adipose tissues in small quantities.

These brown adipose tissues can be found all over the body in areas like the liver, pituitary gland, bone marrow, placenta, fundic glands in the stomach, skeletal muscle and ovaries.

Action & Mechanism

As we have mentioned above, leptin is a huge factor that control the regulation of appetite and metabolism. Aside from that, it modulates the amount of adipose tissues fatty tissues in our body.

The process by which leptin acts on inhibiting appetite is by acting on specific receptors of the hypothalamus in a way that is stimulatory or counteractive, such as:
Leptin stimulates the production of melanocyte-stimulating hormone which acts as an appetite suppressant.

Neuropeptide Y is a feeding stimulant in the gut and leptin can counteract its effects.

Adandammide is a cannabinoid neurotransmitter which also promotes appetite; again leptin can counteract its effects.

How Does Leptin Help In Weight Regulation?

If you lose fatty tissues, it goes to follow that leptin plasma levels also go down, and therefore appetite is fueled so that the body recovers the lost fats. Along with this, bodily energy expenditure is lessened through a decrease in body temperature.

On the other hand, leptin levels are increased if fat mass is increased; therefore weight loss occurs through appetite suppression. This is how leptin regulates your weight.

Leptin also affect the modulation and regulation of onset of puberty. In the cases of thin women, the onset of puberty for them is much later compared to girls who are heavier.

Further, thin girls sometimes fail in releasing an egg from the ovary, or ovulating, during their menstrual period.

Consuming Foods Containing Leptin

With most medical conditions, you can monitor the level of the needed chemical that can be found in your foods. Unfortunately, consuming foods that contain Leptin will not assist you in the matter of Resistance.

The digestive tract is not able to absorb any form of Leptin to increase your personal levels. Searching for foods that contain it and adding them to your diet will not provide any benefit.

In order to be effective, your body must create its own and respond to it. You do not want high levels in your body; this can increase the resistance and ultimately do more damage to the receptors that trigger you feeling full.

The goal is to teach your body to respond to Leptin, and to do so at a lower level.

What is Leptin Resistance?

Leptin is the hormone that controls metabolism and also curbs your appetite. When your brain reads that there is not enough of this chemical in your body to keep it satisfied, it must get your attention. To do so, your body carries out a series of triggers that create hunger.

Unfortunately, your body cannot pull the Leptin it needs from food, so searching for a food that contains it serves no purpose. Basically, what you eat becomes fat, and the fat produces the chemical, which is then released into your blood stream. Once a certain amount is built up in your blood stream, your brain should turn off the hunger response.

When someone is resistant to leptin, their brain does not turn off the hunger response even when they are full.

When you have an abnormal increase in the level of leptin in your blood stream over a long period of time, your body learns to ignore it, which results in Leptin insensitivity, in the same manner the levels of insulin can be ignored in diabetics. Not everyone creates their own Resistance. Genetics can also cause your body to be less responsive to the levels in your blood, in turn decreasing your metabolism, increasing your food cravings, and causing you to gain weight.

The key is to work with your body to increase the sensitivity to the hormone Leptin so that you are able to maintain a higher metabolic rate and control your appetite, even if the level of Leptin in your blood were to drop.

Body fat causes the level of Leptin in your body to increase. Carrying around more weight over a long period of time allows your body to build up a higher threshold for the hormone. Seems like a catch-22 right? How can you get your leptin hormone levels under control when your brain is telling your body that even though you are unhealthy, the weight you are is the weight you should be?
While there are no foods that your body can draw leptin from, there are foods that you can eat to make your body more sensitive to its own levels.

Leptin Resistance and Diabetes

Studies have shown that people who have Leptin Resistance are at increased risk for developing type II diabetes. It is thought that the correlation is due to increased food consumption. The more food you eat, the more insulin your body has to create to keep your blood sugar at a healthy level.

Repeatedly consuming large amounts of food increases your blood sugar. In doing this, your body learns to accept higher and higher blood sugars, because your pancreas cannot keep up with the amount of insulin that your body needs. Once your body becomes "okay" with a higher blood sugar on a regular basis, it triggers your pancreas to create less insulin to compensate, leaving your blood sugar uncontrolled, and leaving your body in a very unhealthy state.

It is important to note that not everyone who is diabetic will develop Leptin Resistance, and not everyone who is Leptin Resistant will develop diabetes.

Those who have Leptin Resistance develop abnormal amounts of fat mass. This is caused by over-eating dietary toxins like wheat, sugar, frying oils, and other unhealthy foods. As the amount of fat in the body increases, the brain becomes immune to the Leptin in releases. It no longer realizes that the body has taken in enough fat to sustain energy, so more and more fat is allowed through.

If extremely high Leptin levels are constantly soaring through the blood, the brain learns to completely ignore the hormone because it is always there. Over time, Leptin Resistance allows large amounts of free fatty acids to deposit outside of the designated deposit locations into other tissues nearby, where fat cells are not supposed to be. This fat then begins to damage the surrounding tissue.

The longer Leptin Resistance is present, the more fat cells grow and the larger they become. When cells become larger than their cell walls are meant to sustain, they develop an instability and rupture. When the cell ruptures, their contents deposit in the tissue, and the body tries its best to clean them up. Unfortunately, it is not able to clean up all of the dead and dying fat cells.

What is left from the cells sets a condition called lipotoxicity and inflammation. Over time, this toxicity begins affecting the pancreas which results in insulin resistance, or type II diabetes.

Who is Susceptible to Leptin Resistance?

Those who are susceptible to Leptin Resistance are unfortunately some of the same people who are susceptible to developing diabetes.
If you have eaten a diet that is full of processed foods, sugar, and eating unhealthy portions.

Other risk factors include:

Family history of Leptin Resistance
Family history of obesity
Personal history of obesity
A sedentary lifestyle
Eating disorders
Lack of regular exercise
Long term high stress levels

Symptoms of Leptin Resistance

High Body Mass Index
Increased stress
Irritably
Mood swings
Nocturnal cravings of carbohydrates
A large appetite
Over-eating regularly
High triglycerides
High cholesterol
High blood sugar
Thyroid problems
Fatty liver
Fatigue
Insomnia
Allergies
Food sensitivities
Acne
Ovarian cysts
Endometriosis

There are a lot of tests your doctor can do to determine whether or not you are Leptin Resistant. First, s/he will perform a physical examination, and ask you a lot of questions about your eating habits, the way you feel, and they will try to determine whether or not you have the symptoms of this disorder, or if your symptoms fit a different problem.

After your doctor has taken your history and completed a physical examination s/he will then order blood tests. Many of these tests can be used to diagnose other medical problems that have similar symptoms.

The Lab Tests Your Doctor Will Perform

Fasting blood sugar A1C – This test will allow the doctor to determine your average blood sugars over the previous three months. This will show them whether you typically have a higher blood sugar than a healthy person does. The typical AC1 level of a person with Leptin Resistance ranges above 5.6.

Homosysteine and C-Reactive Protein – These blood tests check for cardiovascular disease and whether you are at risk for heart disease. CRP also measures levels of inflammation inside your body. Both heart disease risk and inflammation are indicators of leptin resistance.

Urine Test – Markers in your urine will help your doctor determine whether the proteins in your urine are indicative of leptin resistance.

LDL – LDL is bad cholesterol. Those who have, or are at risk for Leptin Resistance typically have higher cholesterol.

TSH – TSH is sort of a catch-all test. It was once thought that this test could rule out thyroid function disorders. Essentially, those who are Leptin Resistant have thyroid problems attached. However, this test does not tell a physician the level of thyroid hormones being released, only what is in the blood. It does not reveal how healthy your thyroid is.

Ultrasound – An ultrasound test is done on three different areas. The liver typically does not contain any fat. In the body of a healthy person, it is muscle, with a few glands and a vascular system. For a person with Leptin Resistance, an ultrasound will show fat build-up around the liver. The ultrasound technician will also check body fat concentration. Those who suffer from Leptin Resistance develop larger fat cells and fat pockets outside of designated deposit locations.

Women who have Leptin Resistance are more prone to ovarian cysts and cysts inside the uterine wall; this is another location that the ultrasound technician will check.

If your doctor determines that you do have Leptin Resistance, or that you are beginning to develop the disorder, they may prescribe medications to help treat the condition. There are typically two medications that are prescribed for treatment of Leptin Resistance. These two medications are commonly used to treat diabetes andthe excessive weight that comes along with it.

Byetta – A diabetic medication that is injectable. It does have certain restrictions and should not be used in combination with certain drugs or disorders. It is commonly prescribed as an "off label" medication to treat Leptin Resistance.

Symlin – An injectable medication used to treat diabetes. However, it can be used off label to help reduce weight and fat in those who have Leptin Resistance.

Even though these medications are authorized for treatment of diabetes, they can be prescribed "off label" to treat Leptin Resistance. The two medications are both used to treat diabetes, but they are also showing a lot of promise in treating the non-diabetic population in stimulating weight loss in those who are overweight.

It is important to note that these drugs do not actually contain leptin, but are used as weight loss agents which remove excess fat from the body. The purpose of removing the excess fat is to deprive the brain of enough leptin to catch its attention, and reprogram it to the markers found in the hormone.

There are currently no medications that are used specifically for Leptin Resistance. However, there are some changes that can be made in lifestyle and diet that can assist in treating Leptin Resistance. There are also some natural supplements that can be used.

Treating Leptin Resistance Naturally

While there are some medications to treat Leptin Resistance, often the most effective way to treat a problem with the body is naturally. Even if you are on medications prescribed by your doctor, taking a natural approach alongside treatment can improve the outcome of your situation and allow you to gain faster control of your situation.

Exercise

While the prescription medications that are given for Leptin Resistance are aimed at treating the associated weight gain, they are not able to reverse it, or to treat the underlying issue. Since Leptin Supplements do not help, due to your digestive system being unable to extract this chemical from your daily intake, exercise becomes one of the most effective treatments for Leptin Resistance.

Exercise helps reduce Leptin Resistance by increasing serotonin levels in the brain and by burning the excess fat that your brain is ignoring. Burning this fat allows your leptin levels to come down. This may make you feel hungry more often, and may make you want to eat more. However, following a diet plan can help you lose weight, and take control of your leptin levels as well.

The key to treating leptin is to slowly allow your brain less and less Leptin, and bring it back in tune to the chemical in general. For a long time, your brain has been ignoring the levels of Leptin coursing through your blood stream. Once you begin depriving it of Leptin, it will take notice that there has been a major change, and over time, it will adjust to lower and lower levels of this hormone.

If you are not able to withstand high impact exercise, such as cardio, you can start with any exercise. Walking is a great starter exercise. Joining water aerobics will allow you to burn fat without damaging your joints or causing yourself any undue pain.

Keeping up on your exercise, and slowly increasing the duration and frequency, will allow you to burn the excess fat that is releasing Leptin into your body.

In order to curb your cravings while you are depriving your brain of high levels of Leptin, you need to have a great diet plan in order, and you need to follow it completely.

Leptin Resistance Diet

There are many foods that you should eat while on a Leptin Resistant diet. There are also foods that you should eat in moderation or not at all while on this diet. Essentially, you are aiming for a low fat, low cholesterol, low carbohydrate, and high protein diet.

There is a cheat sheet at the end of this book that contains three tables.

The first table is foods you should focus on. The second table is foods you should avoid for the first three weeks of your diet, and the third table contains foods you should avoid completely to reduce your Leptin Levels.

Your diet should contain at least 1,200 calories per day. No matter how desperate you are to lose weight and take back control of your life, you should never consume less than 1,200 calories per day.

You should try to focus mostly on plant-based foods throughout the day. Snacking on vegetables is a great way to curb cravings and to manage your caloric intake, especially if you are used to taking in larger amounts of food than the recommended serving size.

Tips for Cooking

Vegetables

Vegetables have the most nutritional value when they are raw. Once they are cooked, they tend to lose a lot of the benefits they provide to your body. Vegetables should be steamed, and only cooked enough to bring out their flavor. The best way to cook them is through steaming and not through boiling, sautéing, or microwaving. These methods will over-cook the vegetable and will reduce the nutritional value.

Cooked vegetables should not be mushy. Vegetables that still retain resistance when you bite into them take longer to digest, which in turn keeps you full longer.

Meats

Red meats should be cooked to medium well and should never be well done. This is because beyond medium well, the meat begins to lose nutrients, and the protein levels begin to drop. Chicken and pork should always be well done because they contain more bacteria which can be dangerous to your health if they are not cooked through.
Using a counter top grill can be very beneficial, an outdoor grill is not. Charred foods, while delicious, pose serious health risks and increase your risk of developing cancer. While you are trying to solve one problem, there is no need to create another.

Length of Diet

This diet should not be followed long term. It is a short-term diet only that should be followed for a maximum of six weeks at a time. The diet can be done more than once, but you should always have a 2 week rest period between diet phases. By following a strict diet and exercise regimen, you will be able to reset the leptin receptors in your brain to pay more attention to the levels in your blood.

Healing your body from Leptin Resistance does not just include physically healing. It includes emotional healing as well. It involves finding inner peace and finding a new you. This can be a very emotional time in your life, and making sure that you have the right support system is very important.

There are many things that you can do to ensure that you are healing yourself as a whole. Meditation, acupuncture, massage, reflex therapy, and sometimes counseling may be necessary to help you along your journey to finding a new you.

Meditation

Stress can increase the urge to eat, increase the amount of leptin in your blood, and increase your blood pressure. It is very important that you take time to rid your body of stress and feel better about yourself.

Meditation is great for your health, great for your mind, and great for your spirit. It allows you time to reflect on your emotions and manage them in a healthy way. You can learn to manage the emotions and the way your body feels from day to day.

One of the most important things you can do on your journey to reversing leptin resistance is to pay attention to your body. You are making a dramatic change in your life which can become an emotional roller coaster. It is important for you to manage your emotions as they come, and to not ignore them.

Not only are you healing yourself physically, but you are healing yourself emotionally as well. You are creating a new life, and you are shedding a lot of weight. Coming to terms with the changes occurring in your body can be made a lot easier by creating an inner peace.

Acupuncture

Over the last several years, there have been reports of people overcoming Leptin Resistance with a combination of diet, exercise, meditation, and acupuncture. If you are a believer in natural and alternative medicine, you may find a great deal of benefit in a routine acupuncture visit.

Acupuncture releases negative energy from your body, releases pain, and relieves inflammation.

It can be very relaxing. Since pain and inflammation are major factors in Leptin Resistance, you may notice a substantial change in your ability to get up and move around, which makes exercise easier and less painful.

Massage

Along your journey to find a healthier, smaller you, massage may be extremely beneficial. Exercise can be difficult and very painful if you are heavier and are overcoming years of weight gain.

Massage not only helps relieve pain, but it also makes you feel better about yourself and your ability to overcome your circumstances. Make sure that your massage therapist has worked with people who have had Leptin Resistance or diabetes.

Reflexology

When most people think of reflexology, they think of treatment for the immune system, or even getting reflexology to assist in comfort in the early stages of labor. However, reflexology has much more to offer, especially now that you are going through a total body change. Since excess fatty tissue in the body can cause your immune system to become weak, reflexology is able to help with inflammation and with building your immune system back up while you work on getting rid of the excess weight. You do not have to wait until your transformation is complete to start reflexology. You can begin both your journey and reflexology at the same time.

Supplements for Reversing Leptin Resistance

While there are no supplements containing leptin that benefit the human body, there are some that make it easier to create leptin and process it. These are supplements like omega-3s, dietary fiber, zinc, and melatonin.

Omega-3s – these fatty acids help adjust leptin sensitivity. They help the brain recognize chemicals in the brain at lower levels. You should not ingest too much omega-3 fatty acids. The limit should be no more than 3 grams per day.

Dietary Fiber – Fiber helps break down fat and flush out impurities. It also helps reduce cholesterol and burns fat at a faster rate. While most foods are not a great source of dietary fiber, you can use fiber supplements to increase your daily intake. These supplements can be in the form of capsules, pills, and drink mixes.

Zinc – Zinc is a mineral that helps the brain recognize leptin. It can be taken in the form of a standalone vitamin, or in the form of a multi-vitamin.

Melatonin – Melatonin is a natural sleep aid. It is a chemical found naturally in the brain that helps you fall asleep. Taking a melatonin supplement can increase your quality of sleep.

Getting enough sleep, and enough quality sleep can greatly impact your ability to process certain chemicals in your brain.

Water – While water isn't a supplement, in this case, it can be. A dehydrated body does not burn fat at the same rate that a hydrated body does. Water helps flush away excess chemicals, hormones, and build up from the body. Staying hydrated can dramatically increase your ability regulate your leptin levels.

The Low- Down on Leptin

Now that you have an overview of what leptin is and how to go about the Leptin Diet, let us now go deeper into the realm of leptin. In this section you will learn about the many benefits that you can have from this type of diet.

Further on, you will be introduced to the Venus Factor concept and its relationship to the Leptin Diet. Lastly, you will also learn about the important food components within the diet.

Pro & Cons of The Leptin Diet

The discovery of the hormone leptin in 1994 has caused medical researchers a lot of excitement because there is finally a way to explain how this hormone affects our food intake as well as body fats.

Although it has been more than two decades, the study of leptin when it comes to weight loss is not extensively studied. Nevertheless, there are some studies that have pointed out the advantages and disadvantages of this particular diet program.

The Advantages

Leptin is characterized as a high protein diet. The biggest advantage of eating a high protein diet is that it leaves you feeling more full and satiated, compared to when you eat more carbohydrate-rich foods. The reason for this is that protein seems to be digested slower than carbohydrates.

Since you feel satiated for a long time with high protein diet, you also do not need to eat frequently, thus you use up and burn excess calories and fats respectively resulting in weight loss.

The Disadvantages

Just like any other type of diet regimen, the Leptin Diet also comes with several disadvantages. Although people lose weight from the Leptin Diet, most of it is water weight. Eating a high protein diet forces the human body into starvation, which results in the cells running out on glucose.

When there are not enough carbohydrates to be converted into blood sugar, the muscles deteriorate and leak water. If not properly addressed, this can lead to irritability, headaches and an overactive kidney; which can possibly lead to cardiac arrest.

On the other hand, a high protein diet is also high in saturated fats. Increasing the fat intake also puts dieters at risk to heart diseases as well as stroke. Lastly, a high protein diet lacks the necessary nutrients required by the body in order to function properly.

This is the reason dieters who opt for this particular diet program are encouraged to take in supplements to compensate for the nutrients that they cannot get from protein.

Maintaining Proper Levels of Leptin

In the previous section, it was discussed that leptin is a hormone that is naturally occurring in the body. Moreover, there are some things that counteract with this hormone, including fats. In fact, more fat in your body results in leptin resistance thus making it hard for you to feel satisfied and satiated, even after a full meal.

Maintaining a good level of leptin is very important for your metabolism. However, there is really no effective way of measuring the exact levels of leptin in the body. Although this may be the case, there are markers that are used in order to determine your leptin resistance levels. Taking the test will help you determine what course of action you should take in order to increase its level for the sake of your metabolism.

Below are some tests that you can do to find out if your leptin levels are okay.

Have your blood sugar taken after fasting for at least 12 hours. If you get a reading above 95mg/dL, then it is likely you have leptin resistance.

Take the AC1 test for your blood sugar and if the value is above 5.6 then you are likely to be leptin resistant.

Have your cholesterol and triglyceride levels checked as leptin resistance is linked to high levels of LDL.

Undergo an ultrasound to find out if you have fatty liver is also a sign that you are leptin resistant.

On the other hand, you can also check for physical signs to find out if you are leptin resistant. One of the best indicators is your weight, and if you are obese or suffering from diabetes, then you are likely to suffer from leptin resistance.

Other physical signs that indicate leptin resistance include fatigue, high blood pressure and the presence of stretch marks and skin discolorations. Having low levels of leptin in the body can sabotage your metabolism.

Here are some tips on how you can maintain the right levels of leptin in your body.
Get Enough Sleep. It is important to get at least six to eight hours of restful sleep during the evening. Aside from allowing your body to repair itself, sleeping also subjects you to involuntary fasting which allows your body to produce more leptin.

Avoid High Fatty Foods. Eating foods that are fatty as well as salty can make you leptin resistant. Although the Leptin Diet requires you to eat protein, which also comes with a certain amount of fat, eating lean meats is your best option. Getting your daily amount of fibers and carbohydrates will also help you flush out the fats from your body.

Exercise. Regular exercise can help boost your body's metabolism. It will help improve how your body utilizes leptin. Moreover, exercise also helps to burn your body fat. The lower your body fat, the more leptin your body produces.

You really do not need to take anything in order to maintain the proper levels of leptin in your body. It is necessary to maintain a proper lifestyle; eat healthy and exercise regularly.

Venus Factor & Leptin Connection

There are two important hormones that control metabolism. The first is insulin, which is the hormone that breaks down carbohydrates (sugar) to be used as energy by the body. The presence of a high amount of insulin in the blood stream indicates that your body is able to convert a lot of sugar into fats.

Another underrated and recently discovered hormone that influences the metabolism of the body is leptin. Unlike insulin, the presence of high levels of leptin is good because it gives the metabolism a good kick. However, leptin can easily inactivate if the body has a high amount of stored fat. This is the reason why high levels of insulin can contradict the action of leptin.

Leptin resistance is a big problem among many women because women are hardwired to store more body fat than men due to reproductive evolution. This is the reason women tend to have slower metabolism than men.

Although women tend to be leptin resistant, there are ways to correct this. One of the solutions is the Venus Factor Diet, developed by John Barban with the collaboration of Brad Pilon and Brad Howard.

Understanding the Venus Factor Diet

Women tend to eat what they want without any regard to the physiological needs of their bodies. The program focuses more on the right nutritional path that women should take in order to decrease their insulin levels and increase the leptin levels in their bodies. This particular weight loss system is an updated version of the Venus Index Program.

The Venus Factor Diet is a program that emphasizes on correcting the diet of women, while the latter focuses on teaching women an exercise regimen that will help them shed off their body fat fast. Since the Venus Factor Diet is the updated version of the Venus Index, it also covers most of the effective exercise regimen of the previous program.

What Is Included In the Venus Factor

When you get the Venus Factor Diet, you will also receive an exercise manual that will teach you how to tone and sculpt your muscles. Sculpting your muscles is very crucial in weight and fat loss because it helps improve the metabolism of the body.

Moreover, you will also get a nutritional guide on how to feed your body right so that you can lose your excess pounds without crashing your metabolism. You will also get the 12-week fat loss system book to keep you informed as well as track your progress while doing the program.

Basically, the Venus Factor serves as your guide or manual on how to do things properly to boost the metabolism as well as maintain the right hormonal balance in your body.

What Can You Eat?

The aim of the Leptin Diet is to reduce hunger and prolong the satiated feeling. This can only be achieved by eating the right kinds of foods.

The Leptin Diet is famous for being high in protein foods, but this does not mean that you are restricted purely to eating protein. Below is a food guide for what you can eat and what foods you should avoid when following this particular diet.

Fish

Fish is a good source of leptin. Healthier options for fish include halibut, cod and salmon. Aside from being a good source of lean protein, fish is also a good source of omega-3 fatty acids. You should avoid catfish because they tend to have a higher fat content than other fishes.

Lean Meats

Lean meats from chicken breasts and lean cut are great for your leptin diet, because the Leptin Diet suggests that you eat foods that are high in protein more than anything else. Other sources of lean proteins include spirulina and vegetable protein.

Beans

Beans can help your body maximize your leptin use. Beans do not only contain protein, but also contain fiber, which can make us feel full faster. Examples of beans that you can include in your leptin diet include kidney beans, pinto, lima, lentils and soybeans.

Raw Vegetables

Raw vegetables should also be included in your Leptin Diet because they help your body to fully utilize leptin. Moreover, raw vegetables contain low calories and they are also jam-packed with a lot of fibers to keep you feel full faster.

Examples of vegetables that you should include in your diet are carrots, cucumbers, beets and celery. Berries and fruits are also necessary in the Leptin Diet.

The diet is all about eating healthy and avoiding high fats and sweet foods. Moreover, it is also very important that you chew your food slowly so that you can give the leptin time to work and signal your brain that your stomach is full.

The Concept Behind The Diet

Leptin has been given a lot of attention among those who want to lose weight. What makes leptin very promising among dieters is that it has the ability to regulate the appetite as well as the metabolism of fats.

The concept of the Leptin Diet is based on improving the amount of this naturally occurring hormone in our bodies to make us lose weight. But before we delve deeper into this, it is important to understand the five basic rules of the Leptin Diet to understand how it works.

Rule #1: Never Eat After Dinner

In the Leptin Diet, people are discouraged to go to bed on a full stomach. It is important that you allow at least 11 to 12 hours between your dinner and breakfast.
The reason for this is that the leptin follows a 24-hour rhythm and its peak level is during nighttime.

Leptin can only function properly if you do not increase your fat intake at nighttime.

Rule #2: Eat Three Complete Meals Each Day

Some diet regimen would recommend eating small meals constantly during the day. However, the Leptin Diet recommends only three meals every day with no snacks in between meals. Moreover, each complete meal should have at least five to six hour intervals in order to clear away the triglycerides from the bloodstream. The five to six hour interval gives the liver enough time to process the triglycerides in the body. The presence of triglycerides in the bloodstream can clog the entry of leptin to the brain which can cause leptin resistance of the body.

Rule #3: Never Eat Large Meals

When you follow a leptin diet, make sure that you do not eat large meals as this will cause you to become leptin resistant. Eat slowly so that you will be able to feel genuinely full with your food. Eating food too fast gives you the tendency to eat more because your brain takes time to produce the signal that you are already full.

Rule #4: Eat Protein-Rich Breakfast

Most people eat a lot of carbohydrates for breakfast, but those who eat a high protein meal for breakfast can increase their metabolism by as much as 30%. Eating a high carbohydrate breakfast can also enhance the metabolic rate of the body, but by only 4%. Moreover, eating a high protein diet can also make people sustain their activities for a long time even without food. You also have fewer cravings later in the afternoon or in the evening if you eat high protein foods for breakfast.

Rule #5: Reduce Your Carbohydrate Intake

Carbohydrates are important because without them, the thyroid shuts down, the muscles weaken, and the electrolytes get deregulated.

However, many people focus too much on eating carbohydrates, which results in obesity. The Leptin Diet requires you to reduce the amount of carbohydrates that you eat to no more than 50% of your plate.

Moreover, to check if you are eating too many carbohydrates in your diet, weigh yourself before bedtime and the morning after. If the weight difference is more than two pounds, then you are consuming too many carbohydrates in your diet.

By cutting back on carbohydrates, you will give leptin a chance to improve your metabolism so that you will be able to lose weight fast and burn fats easily.

Research regarding the Leptin Diet is still within the infancy stage, but it is gaining popularity because this type of diet regimen is simply convincing; especially among those who want to lose weight in a healthy manner.

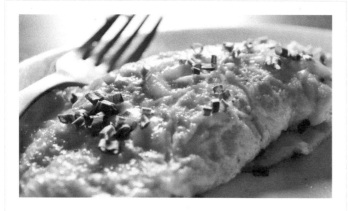

1. Omelet

This omelet breakfast recipe is quick and easy to make. Aside from making that egg dish simply delicious, it also adds something different to your usual egg dish. Serving Size: 2

Nutritional Facts:
Calories per Serving: 511
Fat: 29.5 g
Cholesterol: 105 mg
Carbohydrates: 26 g
Fiber: 7.5 g
Protein: 40.2 g

Ingredients:
2 large eggs
½ pound beef tip
7 baby Portobello mushrooms, sliced
½ onion, sliced
½ red bell pepper, chopped
½ green bell pepper, chopped
2 tbsp butter
Pepper and salt to taste

Directions:
1)On medium high fire, place medium saucepan and melt butter.

2)Sauté mushrooms, onion, and bell peppers for five minutes, or until tender.

3) Add beef and continue sautéing for another 5-10 minutes or until beef is cooked and browned.

4) Meanwhile, in a small bowl, beat eggs, add pepper and salt to taste then pour into saucepan.

5) Let omelet cook until firm, around ten minutes.

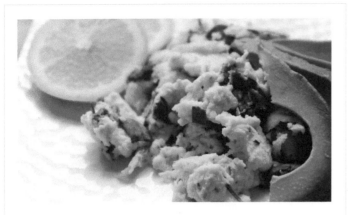

2. Rosemary Eggs

Makes 2 Servings

Ingredients:

2 eggs

½ teaspoon chopped fresh rosemary

3 tablespoons low-fat cream cheese

1 tablespoon fresh lemon juice

1 teaspoon avocado oil

1 teaspoon flax oil

1 ripe avocado

Pinch of cayenne

Salt to taste

2 slices of manna from heaven bread

Instructions:

Mix the fresh rosemary, cheese, lemon juice, avocado oil, flax oil, salt and a pinch of cayenne on a bowl using a fork.

In a deep pan, add about two inches of water, bring to boil then simmer.
Crack the eggs one at a time in a cup and mix then slowly slip the egg mixture into the water as close to the surface as possible. Simmer the eggs for five minutes then remove using a slotted spoon and drain off using excess water.

You can then toast your bread. Cut the avocado into two then remove the seed and cut the meat with the skin on, then scoop the chopped avocado onto your toasted bread. Top the bread and avocado with the poached eggs and cheese mixture.

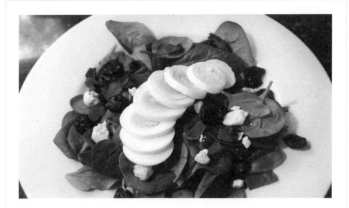

3. Hard-Boiled Eggs With Spinach

Makes 2 Servings

Ingredients:

1 cup baby spinach

2 eggs

3 tablespoons flax oil

2 tablespoons sesame seeds

½ cup chopped fresh basil

1 teaspoon tamari

1 tablespoon flax seeds

Pinch of cinnamon

Instructions:

For the dressing, mix the flax oil, sesame seeds, basil, tamari, flax seeds and cinnamon in a blender. Place the eggs in a saucepan, cover with cold water. Bring to boil and reduce the heat and simmer for 5 minutes.

Fill a saucepan 1/3 full withwater, and bring to a boil then put the spinach and turn down to simmer for five minutes.

Cool the eggs in cold water peel and slice them. Drain your baby spinach and divide between two plates. Arrange the sliced eggs on top of the spinach and drizzle with the dressing.

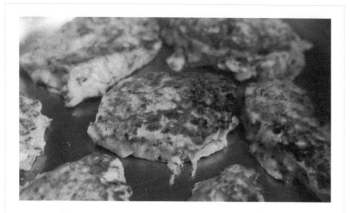

4. Zucchini Pancakes

Makes 1 Serving

Ingredients:

¼ cup fat-free cottage cheese

1 egg white

2/3 cup shredded zucchini

1 tablespoon whole wheat flour

1 tablespoon olive oil

1 tablespoon minced onion

Garlic powder and salt to taste

Instructions:

Preheat a non-stick pan over medium heat. Mix all ingredients in a bowl except the egg white. Beat the egg white until stiff and fold egg into the zucchini mixture.

Spread the batter onto the pan and spread out. Let it cook until batter sets before turning.

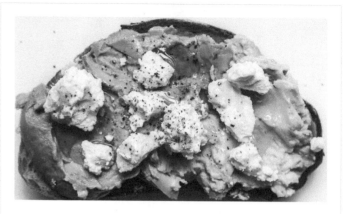

5. Avocado And Smoked Almond Toasts

Makes 2 Servings

Ingredients:

1 ripe avocado

6 ounces smoked salmon

1 garlic, chopped

¼ cup chopped fresh cilantro

2 slices manna from heaven bread

1 teaspoon flax oil

1 tablespoon lemon juice

Instructions:

Put the avocado, garlic, lemon juice, cilantro and flax oil in a blender and blend.

Toast the two slices of bread then add the avocado and top with the smoked salmon.

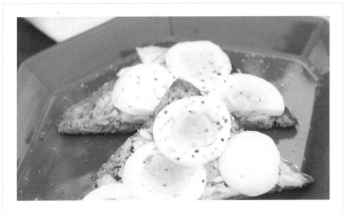

6. Boiled Eggs With Bread

Makes 2 Servings

Ingredients:

2 slices of manna from heaven bread

2 eggs

Pinch of cayenne

Salt to taste

Instructions:

Place eggs in a saucepan, cover with cold water and bring to boil, then reduce the heat and simmer for three minutes.

Cool the eggs in cold water then remove the shells. Cut the eggs into large pieces and put on each piece of bread then sprinkle with cayenne and salt.

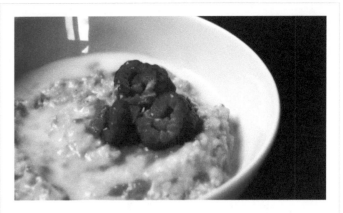

7. Raspberry Vanilla Oatmeal

Makes 2 Servings

Ingredients:

¾ cup uncooked oats

Fresh raspberries to taste

½ cup almond milk

½ scoop of whey protein powder

2 dates blended in water

½ teaspoon vanilla extract

Walnuts or almonds to garnish

A dash of salt

Instructions:

Mix the ingredients except the nuts and refrigerate overnight.

Serve cold or warm and top with the raspberries and nuts.

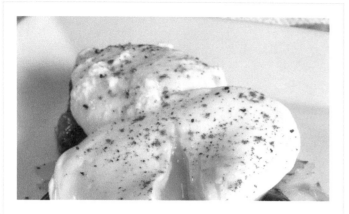

8. Turkey Sausage With Poached Eggs

Makes 2 Servings

Ingredients:

2 turkey sausages

2 poached eggs

Pinch of cayenne

Salt to taste

Instructions:

Broil the sausages for five minutes on each side, blot excess oil with paper towels and put on a plate.

Top with poached eggs sprinkled with eggs and cayenne pepper.

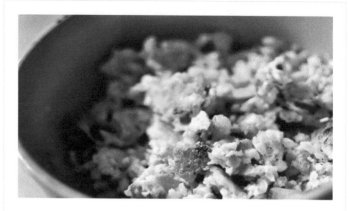

9. Scrambled Tofu

Makes 4 Servings

Ingredients:

1 lb firm tofu

½ teaspoon turmeric

2 tablespoons nutritional yeast

2 teaspoons low sodium tamari

1/8 teaspoon black pepper

1/8 teaspoon cayenne pepper

½ bell pepper diced

1 broccoli stalk, chopped

½ onion diced

1 tablespoon canola oil

2 slices bacon

Instructions:

Drain the tofu and cut into small pieces in a mixing bowl. Add the tamari, turmeric, yeast, pepper and cayenne. Using a fork mash it all up until there are no large chunks; you can use this immediately or cover with plastic wrap and refrigerate overnight.

Heat the canola oil in a frying pan then add the bacon and sauté until brown and crispy. Add the vegetables and stir-fry until tender. Finally, add the tofu mixture and stir-fry until the tofu is heated through.

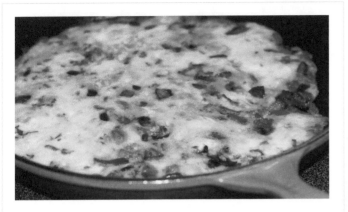

10. Mushroom And Onion Frittata

Makes 2 Servings

Ingredients:

1 lb sliced fresh mushrooms

3 tablespoons butter

1 red onion, chopped

1 shallot, chopped

3 tablespoons olive oil

¼ cup shredded feta cheese

¼ cup shredded Parmesan cheese

8 eggs

¼ teaspoon pepper

¼ teaspoon salt

Instructions:

Sauté mushrooms, onions and butter in oil in an oven-proof pan. Reduce heat to medium and cook for 20 minutes until golden brown while stirring occasionally.

Add the garlic and shallot and cook for one minute longer. Reduce the heat then sprinkle the cheeses and then whisk the eggs, salt and pepper in a bowl and pour on top. Cover and cook for five minutes until eggs are set.

Uncover the skillet and cook for 3-4 minutes or until eggs are completely set. Allow it to cool for five minutes then cut into wedges.

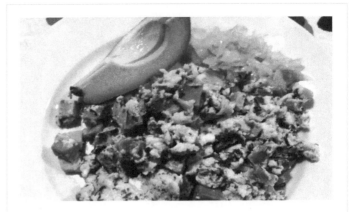

11. Avocado And Ham Scramble

Makes 4 Servings

Ingredients:

8 eggs

1 teaspoon garlic powder

¼ cup fat-free milk

¼ teaspoon pepper

1 tablespoon butter

1 ripe avocado, peeled and cubed

1 cup cooked ham, cubed

½ cup shredded Parmesan Cheese

Instructions:

Whisk the eggs, garlic powder, milk and pepper in a bowl then stir in ham. Melt butter in a large pan over medium heat. Add the egg mixture and cook until almost set then add the avocado and cheese. Stir and cook until set.

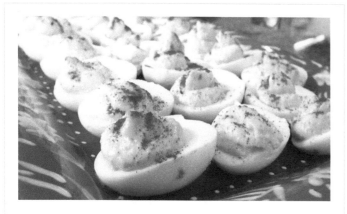

12. Deviled Eggs

Makes 1 Serving

Ingredients:
2 hard-boiled eggs
1 tablespoons non-fat cottage cheese
1 teaspoon chopped parsley
1 teaspoon mustard
Paprika as garnish

Instructions:
Peel the eggs, slice lengthwise, and remove the yolks.

Put the yolks, cheese, mustard, salt, parsley, and pepper in a mixing bowl.

Mash with a folk until blended then return yolks to egg white and garnish with parsley and paprika.

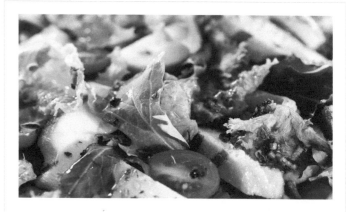

13. Chicken Salad

Makes 2 Servings

Ingredients:
1 boneless, skinless chicken breast
¼ cup chopped walnuts
1 head romaine lettuce, washed and dried
1 ripe avocado
6 Kalamata olives, halved and pitted
For the dressing
¼ cup extra virgin olive oil
1 garlic clove
Salt to taste
¼ teaspoon Dijon mustard
2 tablespoons red wine vinegar

Instructions:
Mix the dressing ingredients in a blender.
Bring 2 inches of water to a boil in a deep pan, reduce to simmer and add the chicken breasts and simmer for 10-15 minutes.

Combine the lettuce, walnuts, avocado and olives in a bowl. Add half of the dressing to the salad and toss well then divide between two plates. Slice the chicken diagonally and arrange on the salad on the two plates.

Drizzle more dressing on each chicken and serve.

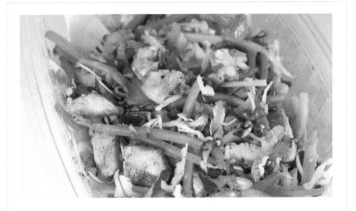

14. Citrus Chicken Salad

Makes 2 Servings

Ingredients:

2 cooked chicken breast halves, cubed

1 cucumber, peeled and chopped

2 celery stalks, chopped

1 tablespoon minced parsley

½ avocado, pitted and chopped

¼ cup chopped walnuts

½ red bell pepper

2 tablespoons chopped cilantro

Dressing

1 tablespoon fresh dill

1 tablespoon olive oil

1 tablespoon minced parsley

3 tablespoons sesame oil

Salt and pepper to taste

Zest of one orange

Instructions:

Mix the walnuts, bell pepper, avocado, parsley, cilantro, cucumber, celery stalks and cooked chicken.

Combine the dressing ingredients in another bowl and mix using a wire whisk.

Pour the dressing over the chicken mixture and store covered in the fridge for a day to let the flavors to blend.

Serve this with a green salad.

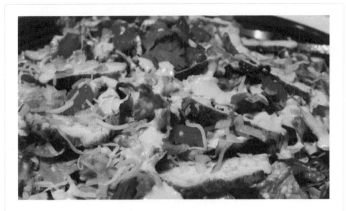

15. Romaine Salad

Makes 3 Servings

Ingredients:

3 cups romaine lettuce, washed and dried

1 celery stalk chopped

½ cup pecans

1 small head radicchio washed and sliced

½ yellow bell pepper, cut into strips

Vinaigrette

¼ cup fresh chopped mint

¼ cup extra virgin olive oil

1 tablespoon lime juice

2 tablespoons lemon juice

Instructions:

Mix the vinaigrette ingredients in a blender. Put the other ingredients in a bowl and pour the dressing. Serve.

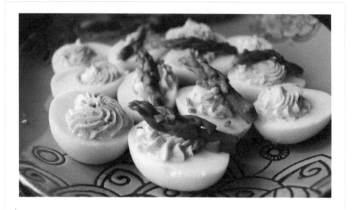

16. Asparagus Soup And Deviled Eggs

Makes 2 Servings

Ingredients:

1 bunch asparagus, chopped

3 cups chicken broth

Salt and pepper to taste

Pinch of cinnamon

¼ teaspoon paprika

2 eggs

¼ teaspoon salt

¼ teaspoon mustard

Salt and pepper to taste

Pinch of paprika

Instructions:

Bring the chicken broth to a boil, add the asparagus, turn down heat and simmer.

Add the cinnamon and paprika and simmer for 15 minutes. Puree the soup in a food processor and add pepper and salt.

Place egg in a pan and cover with cold water then bring to a boil. Reduce the heat and simmer for 15 minutes. Drain and cool the eggs in water then remove the shells.

Slice the eggs in half, gently remove the yolks and place in a bowl then mix with mustard and salt. Mix using a fork and fill the egg whites with the egg yolk mixture.

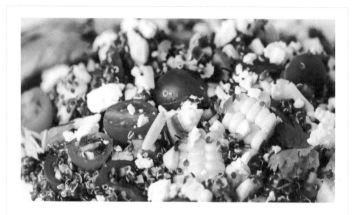

17. Tomato Feta Salad

Makes 1 Serving

Ingredients:

1 carton heirloom tomatoes

Handful fresh basil chopped

1 cup fresh feta cheese

2 tablespoons balsamic vinegar

3 tablespoons olive oil

Salt and pepper to taste

Instructions:

For the dressing, simply mix balsamic vinegar, olive oil, pepper and salt in a bowl then combine the fresh mozzarella, tomatoes and basil. Drizzle the dressing over the salad and serve.

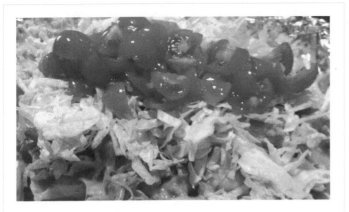

18. Chicken Crockpot

Makes 3 Servings

Ingredients:

3 boneless, skinless chicken breasts

3 shitake mushrooms, stems removed and sliced

1 onion, chopped

2 tablespoons ghee

¼ cup chopped fresh tarragon

5 cups chicken broth

¼ cup chopped cashews

2 bunches spinach, washed

1 tablespoon fresh thyme, chopped

Instructions:

In a large pan, sauté the onion in ghee for five minutes then add the mushrooms and sauté for another three minutes. Add the chicken breasts and brown each side.

Add the herbs and broth and simmer for about two hours ensuring that the chicken is covered with liquid, adding broth when necessary.

Steam the spinach and divide between three plates. Top with chicken breasts, broth and cashews.

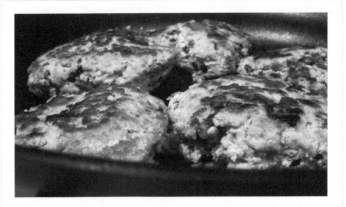

19. Turkey Burger, Mustard Greens And Feta Cheese

Makes 2 Servings

Ingredients:

½ lb ground turkey

2 tablespoons crumbled feta cheese

1 bunch mustard greens, washed and chopped

3 tablespoons ground almonds

1 egg white

Pinch of cayenne

Salt and pepper to taste

Instructions:

Preheat the grill. Mix the egg white, turkey, salt, almonds, pepper and cayenne and form patties.

Fill a large saucepan with water and bring to boil, add the mustard greens, reduce heat and simmer for ten minutes.

Grill the burgers for ten to fifteen minutes on each side until done. In the last few minutes of grilling, top each patty with cheese.

Drain the mustard greens, divide between the plates, top with the burgers and serve.

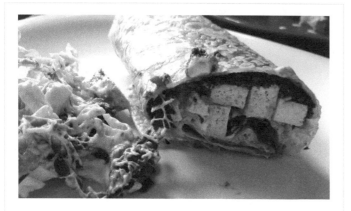

20. Tofu Wrap

Makes 2 Servings

Ingredients:
½ lb tofu

1 tablespoon tamari

2 tablespoons extra virgin olive oil

1 ripe avocado

1 teaspoon lemon juice

1 garlic clove

Dash of cayenne

¼ cup chopped fresh cilantro

1 cup sunflower sprouts

1 cup grated carrots

2 low-carb tortillas

Instructions:
Preheat oven to 400ºF. Cut the tofu into cubes, toss in tamari and olive oil and bake for 20 minutes.

Blend the avocado, garlic, lemon juice, fresh cilantro and cayenne pepper. Spread each tortilla with the avocado mixture. Place the tofu horizontally about 2/3 towards the bottom of each tortilla. Place a line of sprouts and carrots above the tofu and role the tortillas then serve.

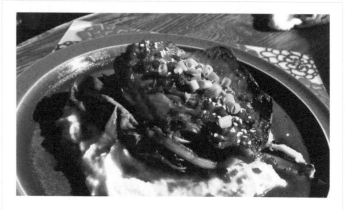

21. Grilled Salmon And Steamed Chard

Makes 2 Servings

Ingredients:
2 (3- ounce) salmon fillets

2 garlic cloves, chopped

2 tablespoons extra virgin olive oil

2 tablespoons chopped fresh parsley

¼ cup lemon juice

1 bunch chard, washed, chopped and steamed

Instructions:
Preheat the grill.

Rinse the fillets and pat dry then rub with garlic and olive oil. Grill the salmon for five minutes each side. Put the chard on a plate, place the salmon, pour the lemon juice, and sprinkle with parsley.

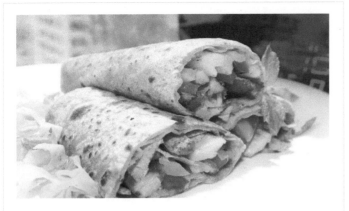

22. Chicken Wrap

Makes 2 Servings

Ingredients:

1 boneless, skinless chicken breasts

2 low carb tortillas

1 tablespoon extra virgin olive oil

Salt and pepper

3 tablespoons chevre

¼ cup sundried tomatoes, chopped

Instructions:

Preheat the grill. Rub chicken with salt, pepper and olive oil then grill the chicken for ten minutes each side or until done.

Slice the chicken, arrange on 2/3 lower part of tortilla, add tomatoes above the chicken, crumble the chevre on top and roll.

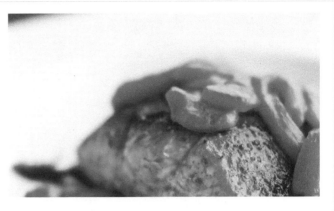

23. Baked Salmon And Asparagus

Makes 2 Servings

Ingredients:

1 tablespoon avocado oil

2 (6-ounce) salmon fillets

¾ lb asparagus

Marinade

½ cup extra virgin olive oil

¼ cup fresh lemon juice

1/3 cup chopped dill

Pinch of black pepper

¼ teaspoon salt

Pinch of cayenne

Instructions:

Preheat the oven to 400ºF. Combine the marinade ingredients in a blender. Place the salmon, skin side up in a glass baking dish and cover with the marinade. Refrigerate for at least an hour.

Bake for five minutes, turn over, and bake for another five minutes.

Fill a deep pan with 1 ½ inches of water. Bring to boil and drop the asparagus. Simmer for five minutes, drain and drizzle avocado oil on top. Add pepper and salt to taste.

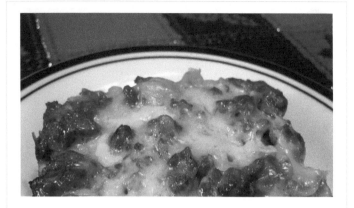

24. Hash Brown & Ham Casserole

Tired of your usual breakfast fare? Add some twist to your ham and hash brown by creating a casserole out of these two main ingredients!

Serving Size: 12
Nutritional Facts
Calories per Serving: 415
Fat: 27.2 g
Cholesterol: 53 mg
Carbohydrates: 29.7 g
Fiber: 2.4 g
Protein: 14.4 g

Ingredients:
1 ½ cups grated Parmesan cheese
2 cups shredded sharp Cheddar cheese
1 container of 16-oz sour cream
2 cans of 10.75-oz condensed cream of potato soup
8 oz cooked and diced ham
1 package of 32-oz frozen hash brown potatoes

Directions:
1) Grease a 9x13 inch baking dish and preheat oven to 375oF.
2) Combine cheddar cheese, sour cream, cream of potato soup, ham and hash brown in a large bowl.
3) Evenly spread mixture into greased baking dish and sprinkle with parmesan cheese.
4) Bake the casserole for an hour or until lightly browned and bubbly.
5) Best if served immediately after baking.

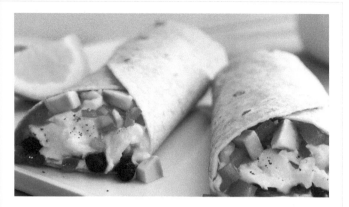

25. Breakfast Burrito

You may not think that a burrito is perfect for breakfast, but it contains healthy ingredients at the right proportions to keep you going until your next meal.

Serving Size: 4
Nutritional Facts
Calories per Serving: 460
Fat: 20 g
Cholesterol: 235 mg
Carbohydrates: 51 g
Fiber: 12 g
Protein: 23 g

Ingredients:
Hot sauce
1 small avocado, 4 oz
1 large tomato, 4 oz seeded and diced
¼ cup salsa
¼ cup reduced fat sour cream
4 pcs of 10-inch flour tortillas
Cooking spray
1/3 cup shredded pepper Jack cheese
4 eggs
4 egg whites
Salt and pepper
¼ tsp chili flakes
1 cup low sodium black beans, drained and rinsed
1 red bell pepper, seeded and diced
½ small red onion, seeded and diced
2 tsps canola oil

Directions:

1) On medium high fire, place a nonstick skillet and heat oil.

2) Sauté peppers and onions for 8 minutes or until onions are soft and translucent.

3) Add red pepper flakes and black beans, cook for 3 minutes.

4 Season with pepper and salt before transferring to a dish.

5) In a separate bowl, beat egg whites and egg until lightly colored and stir in cheese.

6) Place a clean skillet on the fire and spray with cooking spray. Once skillet is hot, pour in beaten egg mixture and cook scrambled eggs, around three minutes. Remove from pan.

7) Spread tortilla on a clean surface, spread 1 tbsp of sour cream, 1 tbsp salsa, ¼ of black bean mixture, ¼ of scrambled eggs, diced tomatoes, ¼ of avocado, add hot sauce to taste and roll burrito and serve.

8) Repeat procedure to the remaining tortillas.

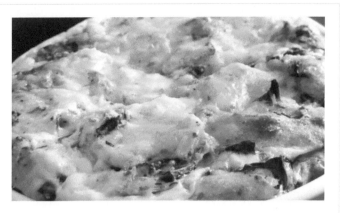

26. Breakfast Spinach & Egg Casserole

You can have all your breakfast ingredients in one convenient dish via this recipe. It's quick and easy to prepare; pop it in the oven and you have a wonderful breakfast meal fit for your Leptin diet.

Serving Size: 8
Nutritional Facts
Calories per Serving: 552
Fat: 38.1 g
Cholesterol: 378 mg
Carbohydrates: 29.9 g
Fiber: 3.1 g
Protein: 23 g

Ingredients:
Pepper to taste
12 eggs, beaten lightly
1 cup shredded cheddar cheese
2 tsp salt
1 onion, sliced
2 tbsp butter
1 pound ground pork sausage
6 baking potatoes

Directions:

1) Grease lightly a baking dish and preheat oven to 350°F.

2) With a fork, prick potatoes and line on baking dish. Cook in the oven for 30 minutes. Remove from oven, let it cool, peel and cube.

3) On medium fire, place medium saucepan and stir fry sausage until lightly browned. Remove from fire and drain oil.

4) In same saucepan over medium high fire, melt butter.

5) Stir fry onions and potatoes for ten minutes until onions are soft and translucent. Season with salt and pepper.

6) Transfer potato into baking dish, top with sausage, cheese, and eggs in that order. Pop in the oven and bake for 30 minutes.

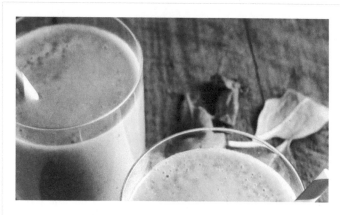

27. Protein Packed Smoothie

If you want to slurp your breakfast, then making a protein packed smoothie is your best resort. This smoothie recipe is nutritious and delicious too.

Serving Size: 1
Nutritional Facts
Calories per Serving: 436
Fat: 11 g
Cholesterol: 0
Carbohydrates: 66 g
Fiber: --
Protein: 31 g

Ingredients:
1 tbsp ground flaxseed
2 cups kale
½ banana
½ cup frozen pineapple
1 cup frozen peaches
1 cup unsweetened almond milk
2 scoops protein powder

Directions:
1) In a blender, mix all ingredients and puree until smooth.

2) Transfer to your bottle and you have a breakfast on the go.

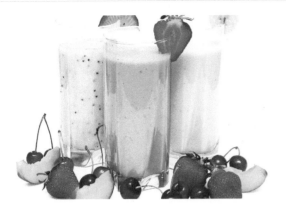

28. Fruity Protein Smoothie

What we love about smoothies is that they are made up of fresh ingredients that are quite nutritious. Plus, it's a great breakfast-on-the-go choice.

Serving Size: 1
Nutritional Facts
Calories per Serving: 349
Fat: 13 g
Cholesterol: 0
Carbohydrates: 45 g
Fiber: 19 g
Protein: 27 g

Ingredients:
1 tbsp Chia seeds
2 scoops protein powder
½ cup frozen mango
½ cup frozen blueberries
1 cup unsweetened almond milk
1 cup spinach

Directions:
1) In a blender, combine all ingredients and puree until smooth.

2) Transfer to a drinking container and enjoy right away.

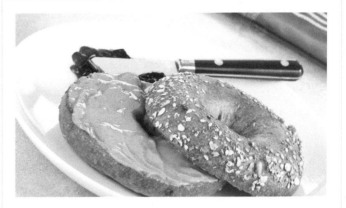

29. Protein Packed Breakfast Bagel

In a Leptin Diet, you are cautioned not to eat too many starchy foods like pasta, bread, rice and the likes. But, you are not entirely discouraged from doing so. So, once in a while, enjoy your favorite sandwich too.

Serving Size: 6
Nutritional Facts
Calories per Serving: 470.9
Fat: 20.7 g
Cholesterol: 221.6 mg
Carbohydrates: 51.0 g
Fiber: 2.2 g
Protein: 19.6 g

Ingredients:
½ cup cheddar cheese, grated or any cheese you like
6 eggs
6 pieces bacon
¼ cup butter
6 miniature whole wheat bagel

Directions:
1) Slice whole-wheat bagels in half. Slather each inner half with butter and set aside.

2) In a greased microwave safe dish, beat eggs season with pepper and salt. And microwave for 3-4 minutes until cooked. Divide cooked eggs into 6 pieces.

3) Crisp fry bacon and half each strip.

4) To assemble, place egg on top of buttered side of bagel, cover with cheese, top with bacon and cover with the other half of the bagel. Serve and enjoy.

5) You can toast bagels prior to assembly.

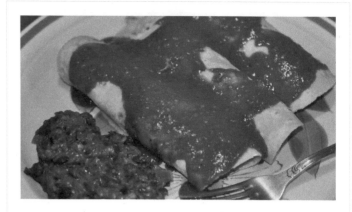

30. Ground Pork Enchiladas w/ Mole Sauce

Tired of the same breakfast day in and day out? Well, try this easy to make ground pork enchiladas to spice up your day.

Serving Size: 8

Nutritional Facts

Calories per Serving: 434.6 g

Fat: 197

Cholesterol: 69.8 mg

Carbohydrates: 34.6 g

Fiber: 2.1 g

Protein: 24.2 g

Mole Sauce Ingredients:

¼ tsp pepper

½ tsp salt

½ tsp ground cumin

1 tsp sugar

1 oz semisweet baking chocolate

1 can of 14.5 oz diced tomatoes with mild green chilies

½ cup chicken broth

Enchilada Ingredients:

½ cup mozzarella cheese, shredded

½ cup Colby-Monterey jack cheese

8 pcs of 8-inch flour tortillas

1/8 tsp ground red pepper

1 lb ground pork, cooked

¼ cup small onion, finely chopped

3 tbsp butter

Directions:

1) Grease a 13x9 baking dish and preheat oven to 3500F.

2) In a 2 quart saucepan, mix all mole sauce ingredients and bring to a boil. Remove from fire and let cool slightly.

3) Transfer slightly cooled mole sauce to blender and puree until smooth and set aside.

4) On medium high fire, place nonstick skillet with butter. Once hot, sauté onion until soft and translucent.

5) Add red pepper, ground pork and ½ cup mole sauce. Stir fry for 3 minutes. Remove from fire.

6) Evenly spread ground pork mixture in the middle of each tortilla.

7) Roll tortillas and place on greased dish with seam side facing down. Repeat process until all tortillas are on dish.

8) Pour remaining sauce over tortillas and top with cheeses.

9) Bake for 20-25 minutes and serve while hot.

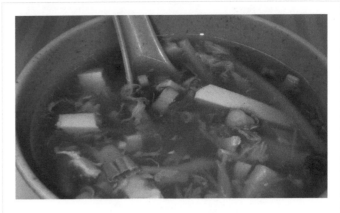

31. Chicken Hot 'N Sour Soup

Hot and sour soup is a renowned Asian dish that many people love. Now you don't have to go to Asian restaurants to enjoy it. Just make it in your home with this recipe!

Serving Size: 4
Nutritional Facts
Calories per Serving: 203
Fat: 7.3 g
Cholesterol: 111 mg
Carbohydrates: 8.4 g
Fiber: 1.1 g
Protein: 25.9 g

Ingredients:

1 egg beaten
2 tbsp cornstarch
3 tbsp red wine vinegar
2 green onions, chopped
1 tbsp sesame oil
1 lb skinless, boneless chicken breast halves, cut into thin strips
¼ tsp red pepper flakes
2 tsps soy sauce
2 cloves garlic, crushed
3 slices fresh ginger root
½ cup sliced bamboo shoots, drained
2 cups sliced fresh mushrooms
½ cup water
3 cups chicken broth

Directions:

1) Mix hot pepper flakes, soy sauce, garlic, ginger, bamboo shoots, mushrooms, water and chicken broth in a saucepan and bring to a boil. Once boiling, reduce fire and let it simmer while covered as you prepare the other ingredients.

2) In a bowl, mix sesame oil and chicken slices. Mix well.

3) In another bowl, mix vinegar and cornstarch then set aside.

4) Increase the fire and bring pot to a boil. Add chicken and slowly pour the beaten egg as you stir the soup.

5) Next, pour in vinegar mixture and continue to stir the soup. Continue cooking until chicken is cooked, around five minutes.

6) Serve hot and garnish with green onions.

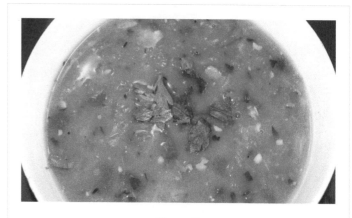

32. Pea Soup

Peas are a great source of protein with less cholesterol and fat. So here's to a hearty soup of pea. You can pair this with a serving of fresh green salad.

Serving Size: 4
Nutritional Facts
Calories per Serving: 195
Fat: 10.3 g
Cholesterol: 31 mg
Carbohydrates: 20.2 g
Fiber: 5.7 g
Protein: 6.8 g

Ingredients:
3 tbsp whipping cream
Salt and pepper to taste
3 cups fresh shelled green peas
2 cups water
2 medium shallots, finely chopped
2 tbsp butter

Directions:
1) On medium high fire, place a heavy bottomed pot and melt butter. Stir fry shallots for 3 minutes or until soft.

2) Add peas and water. Season to taste and bring to a boil. Once boiling, reduce heat to a simmer and cook peas for 12-18 minutes or until tender.

3) Once peas are tender, remove from fire and let cool a bit before transferring mixture to a blender and puree until smooth.

4) Return pureed peas into pot and reheat.

5) Add cream, if using, and season to taste again before serving.

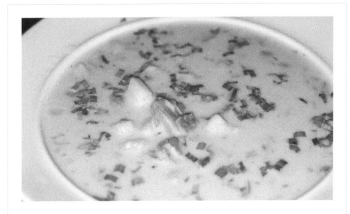

33. New England Clam Chowder

Well, who doesn't love clam chowder? But, did you know that making clam chowder is quick and easy? So, here's our rendition of the famous New England clam chowder!

Serving Size: 8
Nutritional Facts
Calories per Serving: 194
Fat: 5.4 g
Cholesterol: 32 mg
Carbohydrates: 23.7 g
Fiber: 1.4 g
Protein: 12.3 g

Ingredients:
½ cup half and half
¼ cup all-purpose flour
2 cups 2% reduced-fat milk
1 bay leaf
3 parsley sprigs
¼ tsp black pepper
1 ½ tsp chopped fresh thyme
3 cups cubed red potato
1 garlic clove, minced
1 cup chopped celery
1 cup chopped onion
4 bacon slices
2 bottler of 8-oz clam juice
4 cans of 6.5-oz chopped clams, undrained

Directions:

1) Drain clam while ensuring that juice is reserved and combined with clam juice.

2) On medium high fire, place a Dutch oven and crisp fry bacon. Remove and crumble bacon, set aside. Set aside 2 tsp of bacon drippings from Dutch oven and discard the rest.

3) Continue heating the Dutch oven and sauté garlic, celery and onion for 8 minutes or until soft.

4) Pour clam juice and add bay leaf, parsley, thyme and potato bringing mixture to a boil.

5) Once boiling, reduce heat to a simmer. Cover and cook until potatoes are tender, around fifteen minutes.

6) In a bowl, whisk flour and milk until smooth. Pour into pot.

7) Add half and half and clams, continue cooking and stirring for 5 minutes.

8) Discard bay leaf and remove pot from fire.

9) Transfer to serving bowls and garnish with bacon.

10) Serve and enjoy.

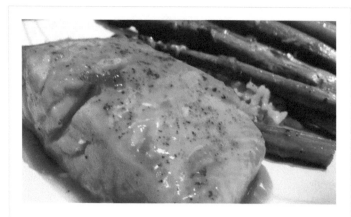

34. Seared Salmon with Roasted Asparagus

Salmon is definitely loved by a lot of people. But, did you know that creating salmon dishes such as this one is quick, easy and delicious? So, try this one out!

Serving Size: 2
Nutritional Facts
Calories per Serving: 405
Fat: 26.6 g
Cholesterol: 104 mg
Carbohydrates: 4 g
Fiber: 1.6 g
Protein: 36.2 g

Ingredients:

2 tbsp grated parmesan cheese
1 tbsp olive oil
1 tomato, thinly sliced
1 tbsp dired basil
2 pcs of 6-oz boneless salmon fillets

Directions:

1) Line a baking sheet with greased foil and preheat oven to 375oF.

2) Place the fillets on the foil, drizzle with olive oil, sprinkle with Parmesan and basil then cover with tomato slices.

3) Pop into the oven and bake for 20 minutes or until cooked and cheese is lightly browned.

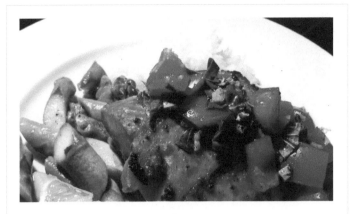

35. Salmon w/ Basil & Tomatoes

Salmon is definitely loved by a lot of people. But, did you know that creating salmon dishes such as this one is quick, easy and delicious? So, try this one out!

Serving Size: 2

Nutritional Facts

Calories per Serving: 405

Fat: 26.6 g

Cholesterol: 104 mg

Carbohydrates: 4 g

Fiber: 1.6 g

Protein: 36.2 g

Ingredients:

2 tbsp grated parmesan cheese

1 tbsp olive oil

1 tomato, thinly sliced

1 tbsp dired basil

2 pcs of 6-oz boneless salmon fillets

Directions:

1) Line a baking sheet with greased foil and preheat oven to 3750F.

2) Place the fillets on the foil, drizzle with olive oil, sprinkle with Parmesan and basil then cover with tomato slices.

3) Pop into the oven and bake for 20 minutes or until cooked and cheese is lightly browned.

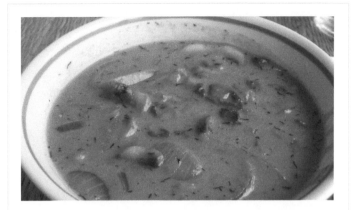

36. Mushroom Soup Hungarian Style

This mushroom soup does not have an overpowering mushroom flavor. Instead, it has the right balance of spices, making it flavorful. Try it so you'll see what I mean.

Serving Size: 6

Nutritional Facts

Calories per Serving: 201 Calories

Fat: 13.5 g

Cholesterol: 32 mg

Carbohydrates: 14.8 g

Fiber: 2.4 g

Protein: 7.5 g

Ingredients:

½ sour cream

¼ cup chopped fresh parsley

2 tsp lemon juice

Ground black pepper to taste

1 tsp salt

3 tbsp all-purpose flour

1 cup milk

2 cups chicken broth

1 tbsp soy sauce

1 tbsp paprika

2 tsps dried dill weed

1 lb fresh mushrooms, sliced

2 cups chopped onions

4 tbsp unsalted butter

Directions:

1) On medium fire, place a large pot and melt butter.

2) Add onions and sauté until soft and translucent, around 5 minutes.

3) Add broth, soy sauce, paprika and dill. Reduce fire and simmer for 15 minutes while covered.

4) Whisk flour and milk in a small bowl until well blended before pouring into pot. Stir pot occasionally and continue simmering for 15 minutes.

5) Add sour cream, parsley, lemon juice, pepper and salt and continue simmering for 3 minutes.

6) Remove from fire and serve.

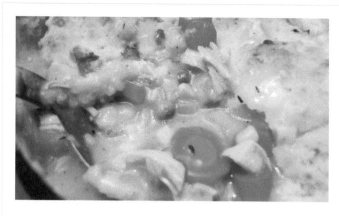

37. Chicken Pot Pie Stew

Making pot pies indeed is hard and cumbersome, but it really tastes good. So, one way you can enjoy the taste of chicken pot pie is to create the filling and forego the pie crusts. Instead, you can easily top your pot pie stew on bread. Easy, easy, right?

Serving Size: 4
Nutritional Facts
Calories per Serving: 263
Fat: 6.9 g
Cholesterol: 37 mg
Carbohydrates: 33.7 g
Fiber: 4 g
Protein: 17.1 g

Ingredients:
¼ of a 16-oz bag of frozen mixed vegetables
¾ tsp ground black pepper
¼ tsp celery salt
½ tsp garlic salt
1 ½ cubes chicken bouillon
½ of 26oz can condense cream of chicken soup
¼ cup chopped celery
¼ of an 8-oz package baby carrots
2 ½ medium red potatoes, quartered
1 large skinless, boneless chicken breast halves, cut into cubes
1 cup water
¼ cup flour
3 tbsp butter
½ of onion, sliced into thin strips

Directions:

1) On medium high fire, place a pot and melt butter. Sauté onions for 3 minutes and add flour. Continue cooking for another 5 minutes, while stirring constantly.

2) Then, add the following: pepper, salts, chicken bouillon, chicken soup, celery, water, carrots, potatoes and chicken. Bring to a boil then reduce fire to a simmer. Simmer for 10-15 minutes while covered or until chicken is cooked.

3) Stir in frozen mixed vegetables and cook for another 5-8 minutes.

4) Add more flour if desired consistency is not attained.

5) Remove pot from fire and transfer chicken pot pie stew into serving bowls and serve.

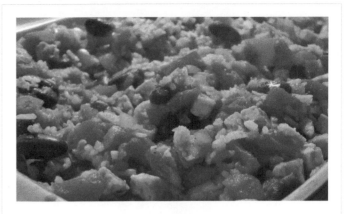

38. Baked Jambalaya

Jambalaya is a Creole dish that is flavorful and considered a classic. Learn how to create this satisfyingly delicious meal at home.

Serving Size: 8
Nutritional Facts
Calories per Serving: 540
Fat: 25.7 g
Cholesterol: 124 mg
Carbohydrates: 47.5 g
Fiber: 2.6 g
Protein: 28.4 g

Ingredients:

2 cups uncooked long-grain white rice
1 ½ cups frozen cooked shrimp
1 ½ cups cooked chicken, cut into bite-sized pieces
1 ½ cups cooked Andouille sausage, sliced
1 ½ cups chopped cooked ham
3 ½ cups chicken stock
1 28-oz can of whole peeled tomatoes
2 tsp Worcestershire sauce
1 tbsp + 1 ½ tsp Creole seasoning blend
1 ½ bay leaves
½ 6-oz can of tomato paste
2 cloves garlic minced
2 stalks celery, chopped
½ large green bell pepper, chopped
½ large onion, diced
¼ cup butter

Directions:

1) Grease a roasting pan without the wire rack and preheat oven to 350ºF.

2) On medium high fire, place a large pot and melt butter.

3) Sauté garlic, celery, green pepper and onion until tender.

4) Add tomato paste, stir continuously and cook for 3-5 minutes.

5) Add Worcestershire sauce, creole seasoning and bay leaves. Cook until heated through and pour into roasting pan.

6) Break tomatoes into pieces by squeezing and evenly put on top of mixture in pan.

7) Stir into pan rice, shrimp, chicken, sausage, ham, chicken stock and juice from tomatoes and combine thoroughly.

8) Cover pan with foil and bake for 1.5 hours. Halfway through the baking time, stir mixture thoroughly.

9) Remove and discard bay leaves before serving

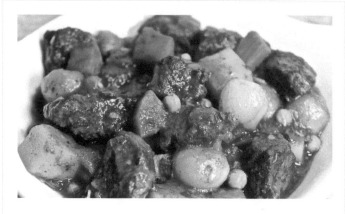

39. Lamb Stew Irish Style

If you need heavy nourishment with less fat and cholesterol content, try this lamb stew. It will give you the protein needed to feed your stamina.

Serving Size: 4
Nutritional Facts
Calories per Serving: 303
Fat: 12.5 g
Cholesterol: 58 mg
Carbohydrates: 27.4 g
Fiber: 4.2 g
Protein: 19.7 g

Ingredients:

1 tbsp chopped fresh parsley, for garnish
2 cups beef stock
Salt and pepper to taste
2 tbsp chopped fresh parsley
1 large stalk celery, sliced
1 carrot, peeled and sliced
1 lb baking potatoes, peeled and sliced
1 large onion, halved and sliced
1 lb cubed lamb meat

Directions:

1) Preheat oven to 325ºF.

2) On an oven safe casserole dish, layer lamb meat, celery, carrot, potatoes and onion in that order.

3) Season with pepper, salt and parsley as you layer the vegetables.

4) Pour beef stock and cover top with foil.

5) Pop in the oven and cook for 1.5-2 hours.

6) Garnish with parsley before serving.

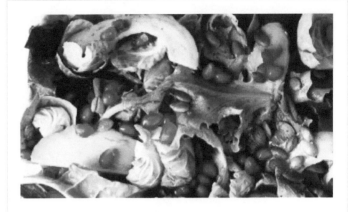

40. Pomegranate-Avocado Fresh Salad

In a Leptin Diet, it is better to eat fruits and vegetables as primary sources of carbs rather than the usual bread, pasta, rice, oats and the likes. Plus, avocadoes will give you the needed protein.

Serving Size: 2
Nutritional Facts
Calories per Serving: 226
Fat: 18 g
Cholesterol: -
Carbohydrates: 16 g
Fiber: 5.6 g
Protein: 2.2

Ingredients:
Salt and ground black pepper to taste
1 tbsp silvered almonds
¼ cup pomegranate seeds
1 cup frisée lettuce
1 ripe large Hass avocado

Directions:
1) Combine oil, maple syrup, vinegar, and pomegranate juice in a container with lid. Shake to mix ingredients thoroughly.

2) Slice avocado in half, discard seed, remove the flesh and cut into ½ inch cubes, while reserving the shells.

3) Then add the cubed avocadoes into the salad greens and toss quickly to coat.

4) Season with pepper and salt.

5) Evenly spread salad into the avocado shell and serve.

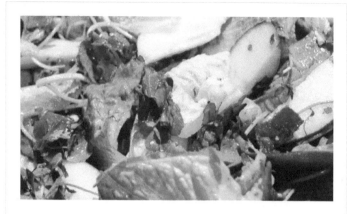

41. Pear & Roquefort Salad

This fresh salad is a great mix of flavors from the sweet and crunchy pecans, fruity taste from pears and tanginess from blue cheese.

Serving Size: 6

Nutritional Facts

Calories per Serving: 426

Fat: 31.6g

Cholesterol: 21 mg

Carbohydrates: 33.1 g

Fiber: 7.4 g

Protein: 8 g

Ingredients:

Fresh ground black pepper to taste

½ tsp salt

1 clove garlic, chopped

1 ½ tsp prepared mustard

1 ½ tsp white sugar

3 tbsp red wine vinegar

1/3 cup olive oil

½ cup pecans

¼ cup white sugar

½ cup thinly sliced green onions

1 avocado peeled, pitted and diced

5 oz Roquefort cheese, crumbled

3 pears peeled, cored and chopped

1 head leaf lettuce torn into bite-size pieces

Directions:

1) On medium fire, place skillet and heat pecans and sugar. Caramelize the sugar and mix pecans. Once sugar has caramelized, remove pecans and let cool before breaking pecans into pieces.

2) Make the dressing by mixing pepper, salt, chopped garlic, mustard, 1 ½ tsp sugar, vinegar and oil.

3) Layer lettuce, avocado, green onions, blue cheese, and pears in a serving bowl.

4) Pour dressing over the salad in the bowl and add pecans before serving.

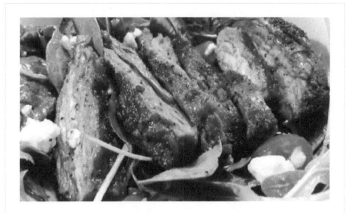

42. Spinach & Steak Salad

This is a great recipe because you are combining a yummy steak into a healthy garden salad. This creates the perfect combination of carbs and protein.

Serving Size: 6
Nutritional Facts
Calories per Serving: 486
Fat: 31.1 g
Cholesterol: 112 mg
Carbohydrates: 12.7 g
Fiber: 3.1 g
Protein: 36.2 g

Ingredients:
½ cup crumbled blue cheese
4 cups baby spinach leaves
½ cup red wine
2 Portobello mushrooms, sliced
3 large red bell peppers cut into ½-inch strips
½ cup Italian salad dressing
1 large red onion, thinly sliced
2 tbsp olive oil
Pepper and black pepper to taste
2 lbs flat iron steak

Directions:
1) Preheat grill to medium high fire and grease grate.

2) With salt and pepper and season the steak. Grill steak into desired doneness. Once done, set aside in a warm area.

48

3) On medium high fire, place a large skillet and heat olive oil. Fry onion until soft and translucent. Add Italian dressing and let boil. Stir in mushrooms and red peppers. Reduce fire and cook peppers until soft around 5 minutes.

4) With a slotted spoon, remove the veggies from skillet and put aside.

5) Increase fire to medium high and pour red wine. For 5 minutes, simmer the dressing until syrupy.

6) In the meantime, divide the spinach leaves onto serving plates. Slice the steak thinly, across the grain and evenly distribute on the spinach leaves. Spoon cooked veggies over the steak and drizzle with the wine sauce.

7) Serve and enjoy.

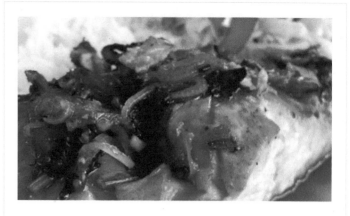

43. Salmon Salad Thai Inspired

Salmon is simply delicious. When paired with fresh garden salad, it brings a special taste to it. Plus, this recipe gives it a tangy flavor with its Thai dressing.

Serving Size: 6
Nutritional Facts
Calories per Serving: 249
Fat: 10.8 g
Cholesterol: 77 mg
Carbohydrates: 11.3 g
Fiber: 2.3 g
Protein: 26.8 g

Ingredients:
1 head lettuce
1 cup chopped fresh basil
1 large tomato, chopped
1 onion, thinly sliced
1 tsp olive oil
1 ½ lbs salmon fillet
4 Thai chilies, chopped
2 tsp brown sugar
4 tbsp lime juice
4 tbsp fish sauce

Directions:
1) Grease a baking tray and preheat oven to 400ºF.

2) Make dressing by mixing chopped chilies, brown sugar, lime juice and fish sauce and put aside.

3) Rub olive oil around salmon steak and place on greased pan and bake for 20 minutes. Once done, allow to cool for 15 minutes.

4) Once salmon has cooled, flake with a fork. Add dressing, basil and tomato. Toss to mix.

5) Place salmon mixture over lettuce leaves and serve right away.

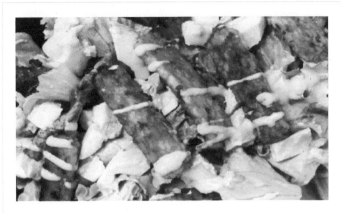

44. Protein Packed Salad

To give you something more lasting, here is a protein packed salad to last you until the morning.

Serving Size: 6
Nutritional Facts
Calories per Serving: 525
Fat: 39.9 g
Cholesterol: 192 mg
Carbohydrates: 10.2 g
Fiber: 4.1 g
Protein: 31.7 g

Ingredients:

1 8-oz bottle of Ranch style salad dressing

3 green onions, chopped

1 avocado peeled, pitted and diced

¾ cup blue cheese, crumbled

2 tomatoes seeded and chopped

3 cups chopped, cooked chicken meat

1 head iceberg lettuce, shredded

3 eggs

6 slices bacon

Directions:

1) Boil eggs. Once cooked, cool, peel and chop

2) On medium high fire, place skillet and crisp fry bacon. Remove from pan, drain and crumble. Put aside.

3) Evenly divide lettuce on to individual serving plates. Layer on green onions, avocado, blue cheese, tomatoes, eggs, chicken and bacon.

4) Drizzle with ranch dressing or any dressing of your choice for that matter.

5)   Serve and enjoy.

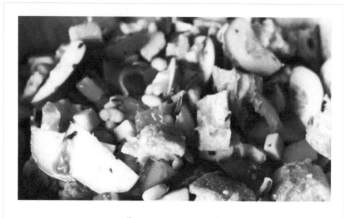

45. Panzanella Salad

Panzanella is a term used for a type of Tuscan salad that is quite popular in summer time. It is usually made of tomatoes and bread.

Serving Size: 8
Nutritional Facts
Calories per Serving: 307
Fat: 21.7 g
Cholesterol: 12 mg
Carbohydrates: 22.2 g
Fiber: 2.1 g
Protein: 6.6 g

Ingredients:

1 cup fresh mozzarella, cut into bite sized pieces

½ cup pitted and halved green olives

10 basil leaves, shredded

¾ cup sliced red onion

4 medium ripe tomatoes cut into wedges

2 tbsp balsamic vinegar

¼ cup olive oil

3 cloves garlic, minced

Pepper and salt to taste

1/3 cup olive oil

6 cups day old Italian bread, torn into bite size pieces

Directions:

1) Preheat oven to 400ºF.

2) In a large bowl mix garlic, pepper, salt and 1/3 olive oil. Add bread and toss to coat. Transfer bread to baking sheet and bake for 5-10 minutes or until golden brown. Let it cool a bit.

3) Meanwhile, mix balsamic vinegar and olive oil.

4) In a big bowl, mix mozzarella cheese, olives, basil, onion, tomatoes and baked bread. Drizzle balsamic mixture, toss and set aside for 20 minutes before serving.

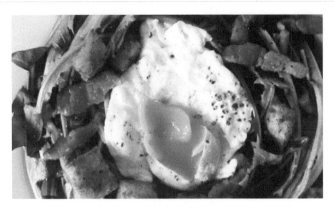

46. Salade Lyonnaise

This fresh garden salad with bits and pieces of protein is inspired by an entry meal salad frequently served in little restaurants in Lyon, France. I hope you will appreciate this delicious salad as much as I did.

Serving Size: 4

Nutritional Facts

Calories per Serving: 709

Fat: 67.5 g

Cholesterol: 227 mg

Carbohydrates: 12.5 g

Fiber: 3.4 g

Protein: 13.7 g

Ingredients:

1 small onion, finely chopped

Pepper and salt to taste

2 tbsp herbes de Provence

1 tsp white sugar

2 tbsp Dijon Mustard

½ cup red wine vinegar

1 cup extra virgin olive oil

2 roma tomatoes, sliced

2 cups curly endive, chopped

2 cloves garlic, finely chopped

1 head romaine lettuce, chopped

4 eggs

1 cup chopped smoked bacon

Directions:

1) On medium high fire, place deep skillet and crisp fry bacon. Drain, place on towel lined plate and set aside.

2) Add 2-3 inches of water and bring to a boil. Reduce heat to a simmer and add vinegar.

3) Crack an egg into a small bowl and hold bowl just touching the surface of simmering water for 2.5-3 minutes until whites and yolks have firmed up but not hard. Remove eggs from bowl and into a warm plate. Repeat process for remaining eggs.

4) On four plates, evenly divide lettuce. Top lettuce with poached egg, bacon, onion, tomatoes and garlic.

5) Make the dressing by whisking pepper, salt, herbes de Provence, sugar, Dijon mustard, red wine vinegar and olive oil. Drizzle on salad.

6) Serve salad and enjoy.

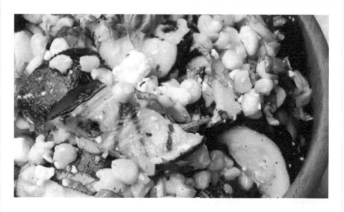

47. Zucchini, Basil & Shrimp Salad

This salad has bright and fresh flavors. It's good to pair this one with a glass of Sauvignon Blanc.

Serving Size: 4
Nutritional Facts
Calories per Serving: 355
Fat: 29 g
Cholesterol: 143 mg
Carbohydrates: 8 g
Fiber: 2 g
Protein: 18 g

Ingredients:

Freshly grated Parmesan cheese, optional

5 oz mixed baby greens

2 cups zucchini, cut into 1-inch cubes

1 lb uncooked large shrimp, peeled, deveined

½ cup chopped fresh basil

½ cup olive oil

½ tsp dried crushed red pepper

1 tbsp Dijon mustard

1 shallot, minced

3 tbsp drained capers

¼ cup fresh lemon juice

Directions:

1) In medium bowl, mix well dried red pepper, mustard, shallot, capers and lemon juice. Mix in basil, oil and season to taste with pepper and salt.

2) In a saucepan with boiling water, add shrimp and boil for a minute. Add zucchini and continue boiling until zucchini is soft and shrimp is cooked.

3) Drain and rinse under cold water, transfer to a bowl and mix in 1/3 cup of dressing, season with pepper and salt. Toss to coat.

4) In a large bowl, add greens and enough dressing to coat. Divide greens into 4 serving plates. Top with shrimp mixture. Place Parmesan on the side.

5) Serve and enjoy.

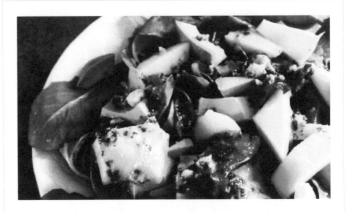

48. Avocado Mango Salad with Chili Lime Vinaigrette

Ingredients:

1/2 jalapeño chili, seeded and minced

Juice of 2 limes

1/4 cup olive oil

1/2 tsp. coarse sea salt

Freshly ground pepper, to taste

1 mango

1 avocado

6 cups organic mixed salad greens

Instructions:

To make the vinaigrette: combine the jalapeño and lime juice in a small bowl.

Whisk in the olive oil.

Season with salt and pepper.

Set aside until ready to serve.

Cube flesh of avocado and mango.

Toss salad greens, avocado, mango, and vinaigrette.

Makes 4 servings.

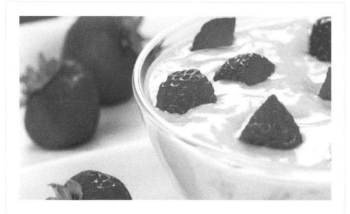

49. Healthy Yogurt Parfait

1 cup Organic Plain Yogurt (antibiotics and hormone-free)

¼ cup Organic Raw Granola (no sweetener)

¼ cup Organic Goji Berries (dried)

Organic Honey, optional, if more sweetness is desired

Instructions:

Add in some of the granola, goji berries, and optional honey to your yogurt, and mix well. Put in serving dish, and top with the rest of your granola and goji berries.

Serves 2.

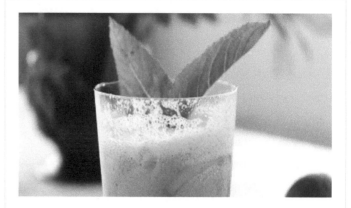

50. Cucumber Mint Cooler

Ingredients:

1 scoop Daily Protein Unflavored

1 cup chopped, seeded and peeled cucumber

1/4 cup chopped fresh mint

1 cup water

1 teaspoon honey

Ice cubes

Instructions:

Combine the ingredients in a blender; process until smooth.

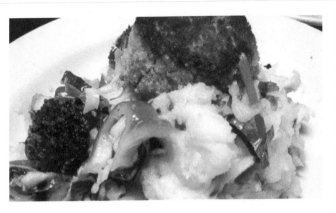

51. Crab and Parsnip in Apple Sauce

Introduction: Crab and parsnip is not a very commonly seen combination. But with a bit of innovation, you may add a zing to normal style of having meals.

Serves: 2-3 persons

Preparation time: 10 minutes

Cooking time: 30 minutes

Ingredients:

1 lb. of crab meat

3/4 cup of parsnip

1 teaspoon of garlic paste

1 teaspoon of cayenne pepper powder

1 medium sized lemon, juice extracted

1 medium sized apple

1 teaspoon of stevia

1 tablespoon of non-fat plain yogurt.

Procedure:

1. Marinate the crab with garlic, lemon juice, and cayenne pepper powder. Keep in this condition for 10 minutes.

2. Pre-heat oven at 350Û Fahrenheit. Place the pork and parsnip inside the oven and cook for 30 minutes.

3. Remove and keep aside.

4. To prepare the apple sauce, peel the apple and boil it. Then add stevia and non-fat plain yoghurt to it. Boil with 4 tablespoons of water to maintain the consistency.

Enjoy the crab dish with apple sauce.

Calorie count: Per serving, the meal contains 510 calories.

Conclusion

Leptin resistance is created when the brain no longer recognizes the chemical hormone leptin in the blood. Leptin is secreted by fat cells. In the leptin-resistant state, the brain has no way of knowing how much fat the body has stored since it can no longer measure the chemical.

Modern medicine cannot reverse this disorder on its own. Even though there are two medications used to help reduce the amount of body fat stored, they cannot make the body more receptive to the chemical itself. The only way to reverse leptin resistance is through diet, exercise, proper sleep, and supplementation.

In order to change your body, you must be willing to change several aspects in your life. You must be willing to change your diet, increase your exercise, monitor the way your body feels, and make adjustments as needed.

The leptin resistance diet is high in omega-3s, dietary fiber, and empty calories. Because of this, you should not follow this diet for a prolonged period of time. The diet should be followed for a maximum of six weeks. If you plan to lose more weight, you should take a two-week break before starting again.

The leptin-resistant diet follows some of the same general principals of a diabetic diet. If you have a confirmed diagnosis of leptin resistance, it is important to be tested for diabetes and other related illnesses, as they are known to coexist.

Did You Like Leptin Diet?

Before you go, we'd like to say "thank you" for purchasing our book. So a big thanks for downloading this book and reading all the way to the end. Now we'd like ask for a *small* favor. Could you please take a minute or two and leave a review for this book on Amazon

This feedback will help us continue to write the kind of Kindle books that help you get results. And if you loved it, then please let me know

Leave a review for this book on Amazon by s earching the title; Leptin Diet 50 Days of Powerful Leptin Diet Recipes to Boost Resistance, Achieve Optimum Health and Lose Weight Naturally!

Check Out My Other Books

Below you'll find some of my other popular books that are popular on Amazon and Kindle as well. Simply click on the links below to check them out. Alternatively, you can visit my author page on Amazon to see other work done by me.

www.ravenspress.com/jjlewisbooks

Dash Diet: Beginners Quick Start Guide to Fast Natural Weight Loss, Lower Blood

Dump Dinners: 101 Fast, Healthy and Easy Dump Dinner Recipes for Everyone

Adrenal Reset Diet: 51 Days of Powerful Adrenal Diet Recipes to Cure Adrenal Fatigue, Balance Hormone, Relieve Stress and Lose Weight Naturally

Mediterranean Slow Cooker: 101 Best of Easy and Delicious Mediterranean Slow Cooker Recipes to a Healthy Life

101 Chicken Recipes: A Mouth-Watering Healthy and Delicious Chicken Recipes that will fill your Stomach

Paleo Slow Cooker: 101 Quick and Easy Paleo Recipes for Healthy Life and Weight

101 Pork Chop Recipes: Extraordinary and Delicious Pork Chop Recipes for Everyday Meals

101 Vegetarian Recipes: Top Vegan Diet Recipes to Live a Healthy Lifestyle

Ketogenic Diet: 101 Days of Ketogenic Diet, Low Carb Recipes for Maximum Weight Loss Benefits

Pressure Cooker Recipes: 101 Mouthwatering, Delicious, Easy and Healthy Pressure Cooker Recipes for Breakfast, Lunch, Dinner in 30 Minutes or Less!

Vegan Cookbook: Vegan Diet for Beginners to a Healthy Everyday Life (Vegan Appetizers and Soups Series)

Paleo Diet: 101 Days of Easy Paleo Diet Recipes Made for Beginners to Maximize Weight Loss

Paleo Diet for Kids: A Fun Pack of 101 Flavorful and Energy-Boosting Paleo Recipes Best In Shaping Healthier, Stronger and Happier Paleo-Nourished Kids

Slow Cooker Recipes: The Best of 101 Nutritious and Delicious Healthy Slow-Cooking Recipes for your Crock Pot

The Juice Cleanse: 101 Healthy Juicing Recipes for Weight Loss

Fast Metabolism Diet Recipes: 101 Best of Metabolism Boosting Recipes to Lose Weight Fast

Low Fat Recipes: 101 Incredible Quick & Easy Recipes for a Low Fat Diet

Gluten Free Diet: 101 Delectable and Healthy Gluten-Free Recipes for better life-style

Diabetes Diet: 101 Healthy Diabetes Recipes to Reverse Diabetes Forever and Enjoy Healthy Living for Life

Wheat Belly Diet: 101 Days of Grain Free Recipes for an Optimum Belly Diet and Weight Loss

Want more FREE Bestselling Cook Books?

Join my **V.I.P** List now!

I will be giving away **Healthy** and Delicious Recipes for **FREE!**

Yes, you heard me right! COMPLETELY FREE to everyone just by being a loyal reader!

www.ravenspress.com/jjlewis/